Genetic Diet

Fat Loss, Energy Gain

By Cathy Wilson

Copyright © 2014

Income Disclaimer

This book contains business strategies, marketing methods and other business advice that, regardless of my own results and experience, may not produce the same results (or any results) for you. I make absolutely no guarantee, expressed or implied, that by following the advice below you will make any money or improve current profits, as there are several factors and variables that come into play regarding any given business.

Primarily, results will depend on the nature of the product or business model, the conditions of the marketplace, the experience of the individual, and situations and elements that are beyond your control.

As with any business endeavor, you assume all risk related to investment and money based on your own discretion and at your own potential expense.

Liability Disclaimer

By reading this book, you assume all risks associated with using the advice given below, with a full understanding that you, solely, are responsible for anything that may occur as a result of putting this information into action in any way, and regardless of your interpretation of the advice.

You further agree that our company cannot be held responsible in any way for the success or failure of your business as a result of the information presented in this book. It is your responsibility to conduct your own due diligence regarding the safe and successful operation of your business if you intend to apply any of our information in any way to your business operations.

Terms of Use

You are given a non-transferable, "personal use" license to this book. You cannot distribute it or share it with other individuals.

Also, there are no resale rights or private label rights granted when purchasing this book. In other words, it's for your own personal use only.

Genetic Diet

Fat Loss, Energy Gain

By Cathy Wilson

Table of Contents

Introduction 9
Chapter 1 – Ancient Days – The Ways of the Caveman 13
Chapter 2 – Factors in Great Health 21
Chapter 3 – Modern Society Living Issues and Science of Living Basics 43
Chapter 4 – Primal Blueprint Factor One: Eating: Take Action Pointers 51
Chapter 5 – Primal Blueprint Factor Two – Exercise – Take Action Pointers 61
Chapter 6 – Primal Blueprint Factor Three – Mental – Take Action Pointers 67
Chapter 7 – Primal Blueprint Factor Four: Social/Lifestyle Take Action Pointers 71
Chapter 8 – Myths of Good Eating and Exercise 75
Final Words 79

Introduction

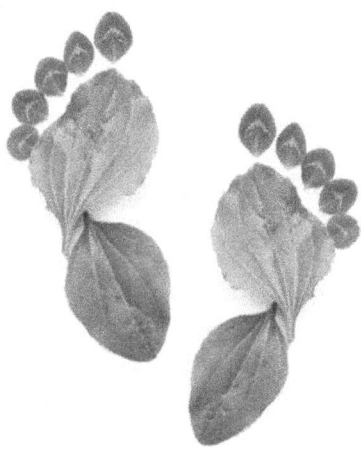

Your mind and body, lifestyle, environment, and social relationships, all influence your quality of life, success, achievement, and longevity. Every choice, action, reaction, inaction, decision, and bouts of luck and hard-luck you encounter, dictate your reality.

Your senses, organs, bones, muscles, nervous system, and internal circuitry, are all tangible factors that evolve over time. These changes are reflective of your actions. From primal to present day, we think, feel, look, act, and respond, differently.

What dictates your basic physiological, mental, social, and environmental needs in the now, is your preset primal blueprint. Your unique genetic coding decides what your body and mind require to function optimally.

These life changing factors we'll discuss, most of us spend a lifetime decoding. Even then, we never figure out everything.

It's safe to say, ancient day man was healthier as a whole, than our societal ways built us today.
Do you only fill your body with organic wild meat, fresh fruits and vegetables, fresh fish and seafood, and crystal clear pure and tasty water?

Not one single bite of disease triggering processed fast food, passed through early man's lips. These people didn't load up on nutrition-less simple sugar pastries, cakes, donuts, and cookies. With short-lived high energy spikes, trailed by deep lows, or deep fried Trans-fat gushing chicken wings or tater tots. Our ancient ancestry never had the opportunity to eat at a gynormous Denny's buffet, or even slather thick rich saturated butter on their daily bread.

Learned unhealthy habits.
Lucky for them, healthy eating wasn't an option!
Unfortunately, we have choice, which ends up causing a lot of preventable heartache, pain, death, and disease. Ultimately, it's the beginning of a faster, more traumatic end, for most.

Is it healthier to rise and fall with the sun, to challenge your lungs and heart every time before you eat, or to stay up late watching TV because you can, skip breakfast, grab a packaged sandwich for lunch, and take-out pizza for dinner, because you're too lazy to cook?
Man used to eat to live.
Now we live to eat.

Intense mandatory interval strength training, and kick-ass cardiovascular exercise was absolute with early man. Every single need a required physical.

The strongest survived.
The weakest perished.
Survival of the fittest was the reality. Harsh, but true, and accepted.
Today we can get by with zero physical conditioning. Excuses take center stage, and slowly but surely, we deny our body its basic intrinsic needs. Over time, we poison our mind and body, from the inside out.

Unknowingly you invite harmful free radicals in, that eventually eat you up.
By allowing this to be your reality, your fate is sealed.
Your only chance is to slow or stop this ticking time bomb, and commit to changing all facets of your health for the better. Shifting back towards the clean eating days. This re-connects emotionally with your mind and body, and removes the toxic interference our society preaches, and makes reality today.

We live for progress, technological advancement, new and more complex in all areas of life, but at what price?
Is your life worth it?
You control **YOU**.
There is no blaming, sob stories, or pointing the finger. Accept and learn from your past. Leave it there, and take action to make your future health all that it can be. Commit to making positive health changes, and you will be rewarded ten times over.
Take my hand, and let's get started.

Chapter 1 – Ancient Days – The Ways of the Caveman

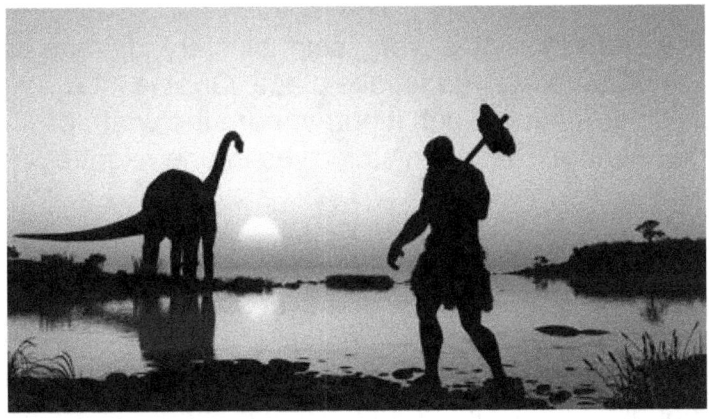

Was it really so simply five thousand years ago, back in the day of the caveman? The time of the Neanderthal might seem totally whacked out crazy. And although there were many hardships, their way of life made sense. People back thousands of years did things because they **HAD** to, not necessarily because they wanted to. Do you really think man wanted to pick up and move whenever Mother Nature threw a natural disaster their way, like drought or flooding?

These harsh elements of nature are what drove their food source away, or destroyed it completely.
There was really no planning back then. They lived reactively day to day.

The necessities of life; food, water, shelter, and health, dictated the way. If there was no food; berries, edible foliage, or game to hunt, the camps had to pick up and move. It didn't matter how blistered and worn their feet were, how achy their backs, or weary their souls were. When water supplies ran dry, there was no choice but to move. The human body can't last more than a day or two without water, even in favorable conditions.

If the weather turned severe; cold, blustery, dry and barren, another move had to take place. Or at least a decision to try and tough it out, or bare the wrath of Mother Nature, that often stole lives in one relentless swoop.

When it came to eating, it was pretty basic. There were no corner stores, freezers, or any sort of convenience that made eating easy. Men had to hunt game, with meat as their main source of fuel; complete protein to provide the nourishment required to build and support lean muscle.

Various berries, herbs, and other foliage, made up the rest of the menu. If the tribe was close to a main water source that had fish, they had the option of adding this omega-rich, and gynormously healthy protective protein to their diet.

That's just about it!

The environment of people in days past, their ability to hunt, pick, and catch food, and the availability of edible food around them, dictated what, and how much they would eat, or if they would eat at all.

They cooked on open fires. Exercise was something they never focused on. Every single thing they did, required incredible amounts of physical exertion.

To say ancient man was mentally and physically strong is an understatement.
From setting up camp and gathering wood to build fires, to hunting game for food and clothing, preparing the food, and making utensils and bowls from which to eat, they had plenty to do in order to eat.

EVERYTHING required exercise. Ancient man had the opposite problem of our society today. They looked for ways to find time to rest their weary bones.

Biological clocks were sharp, because it just didn't work staying up all night, unless you enjoyed sitting in the dark. The only factors that may have routinely interfered with sleep, were either the threat of some sort of attack, or having the duty of caring for the fire.

Everything that went into their bodies was natural. There was no fake interference from external factors, like late night partying and drinking, or crap foods in the wee hours of the morning, because all we have to do is wake up and turn on a light to eat.

Early man didn't have computers and televisions to distract them, interfering with the natural rhythm of the body. When the sun set, it was time for bed. When it rose, our ancestors were up for another day.

Caveman people lived a clean and healthy lifestyle that was tough, but natural.
Caveman Facts

*Proper language wasn't developed. So pictures, gestures, and cave carvings were used for communication. Very few words were spoken if any, more like grunts and grumbles, that we know of anyway.

*Illness and disease that are minor for us today, were often fatal back then. Life was expectancy much lower, where many died before reaching 20 in good times.
*Scientists use the word *caveman,* to describe any type of ancient people.
*Over 200,000 years ago, primitive people appeared on earth – Homo sapiens – the same as you and I.
*Neanderthals are older than *primitive people;* early human ancestors, somewhere around the time of the dinosaurs. They were discovered through fossils, just like the dinosaurs.
*Caveman are often depicted in cartoons, look sort of like apes, hunched over, and very animal-like.
*Caveman died **WAY** before humans appeared.
*These people lived instinctively. When hungry, they hunted for food. If they were cold, they made a shelter, and clothing from wild animals. Our instinctive *fight or flight* response was readily used.

Death often came suddenly and without warning, because of the natural elements of danger from Mother Nature, and the inability to treat most illness and injury. There were no needles to avoid diseases. Skilled surgeons weren't prepped and ready to perform surgeries for serious injuries, except perhaps a few make-shift ones, that were extremely risky back then.

Ancient people were at the mercy of nature, the wrath and the glory.
Factors Caveman Had Right!

EXERCISE
Intense physical activity was something Caveman really didn't have to think much about. There was no need to program a begrudging hour of exercise into the day like

we do. Every single thing our ancient ancestors did required physical effort.

From dawn 'til dusk, the muscles burned, and cardiovascular endurance was challenged. In fact, ancient day people were searching for the opportunity to rest their weary bones, not *treadmill* them.

SLEEP/REST

By the time the sun set hundreds of thousands of years ago, lights were out before the head hit the rock. First off, there really wasn't much to do in darkness, because it was a pain in the butt to make enough light for much of anything. And if firewood was scarce, it would be used sparingly anyway.

Not to mention, these people worked crazy hard to survive daily, and couldn't physiologically do it without a full nights rest, guided by the sun.

The golden ball in the sky was the alarm in the morning, the nighttime signal to get to bed.
Without adequate sleep, caveman instinctively knew they might not have the strength required to ward off their *fittest of the fit* daily life challenges. If they fell ill, the consequence could very well be death.

Caveman couldn't afford to not have adequate rest.
The National Heart, Lung, and Blood Institute states, your brain and emotional well-being can't function optimally with proper rest. Research shows between 7 and 9 hours sleep will suffice for most.
I'm sure ancient man needed more.

THE MENTAL

To say these people took the basics of life seriously is an understatement. Happiness to them, was having enough wild game wandering around to feed the tribe, and rustic supplies to build shelters that served their purpose. Ancient man was thankful when disease wasn't threatening lives, and body injuries were minimal.

HEALTH was priority number one with people of ancient day. Without it, the choice was death.

SOCIAL
Our ancestors lived in families, groups, or tribes for the most part, socially interacting and working with each other as a unit for survival. From as far back as scientists can tell, humans have always needed strong social systems to survive. Outcasts often succumbed to the deathly harsh realities of nature.

Healthy People states, the social factors of good health are in the environment people are born, live, play, work, worship, and get older, which affect numerous aspects of health, function, risks and tolerances, and quality of life. In the olden days, the social was much simpler. Our world has created oodles of stress towards the social, which of course ultimately damages health.

NUTRITION
Caveman didn't live to eat, they ate to live, and survive. Food was a central part of their function. They ate when their body and mind dictated. Like us, primitive man didn't have emotional eating, and habitually snacking. At least to the same degree we do today.

First man, used food as it was intended. To nourish and strengthen the body and mind to perform optimally, fight off disease, and supply the extreme physical strengths required to take care of the essentials; eating, hunting, shelter, making clothing, travel, and building fires, to start.

More often than not, food wasn't readily available. At least not easily accessible when these people were hungry. There was a mind-body challenge for survival, whenever the tummy rumbled.

Experts at *Psychology Today*, states America is the most weight-conscious society on the planet, and the most obese messed up eaters too. Because we are surrounded by food and weight issues, this relentlessly increases our unconscious motivation to pig out.

In Plain English - If you're sitting on a cotton candy couch in Candyland, surrounded by delicious sweets, eventually you're going to want to indulge.
This unstable thought process triggers emotional eating, which is arguably the main culprit for obesity today. But that's another book!

My Thinking…

I'm not saying I want to jump back into caveman days, and live my life clean and free! This would mean giving up my house, toilet, stove, running water, and lights. Convenience does grow on you.
But the way of the caveman, driven without interference through raw instinct, truly is how life should be lived.
Basic Survival Factors:
*Full Bellies
*Warmth
*Water
*Safety
*Shelter

*Avoiding sickness and disease
These were the priority of our ancient ancestors.
Times sure have changed, unfortunately for all the wrong
reasons.

Chapter 2 – Factors in Great Health

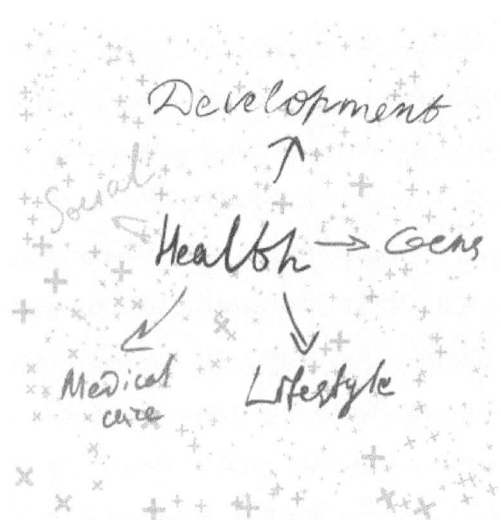

Your health is influenced by numerous factors.
Our focus will be on:
*Diet
*Exercise
*Environment
*Social
*Mental
Some of these factors have changed over the years, while others have remained fairly constant. Heredity, environment, and lifestyle, have stayed pretty much stagnant, as a valued factor in health always, whereas some of the socio-economic factors have developed over

the years, transforming into essential pieces in the master puzzle of great health.

Chalk it up to evolution if you like!

Nutrition, exercise, and socializing, have always held absolute value. Newer on the scene, is education, income, employment, and housing. Caveman really didn't worry about education as we do. The learned their life knowledge by doing.

It's not like they congregated each day down by the stream for classes, that we know of anyway. Typically, the elders taught the younger members of the family, the skills necessary for survival.

Daily living was their education, and employment was life.

Ancient people earned a living building a strong tribe and serving. Another sunrise and sunset was their pay.

Shelter of course was essential, but didn't have an astronomical cost factor associated with it, like it does today. Sweat equity was payment for shelter years ago.

Our society creates stress even when fulfilling our basic needs as human beings. My heart thuds at the thought of even qualifying for a mortgage, or finding a place to rent. Back in the day, caveman simplified the process by picking a spot for their shelter, usually temporary, and physically making it suitable to sleep.

Simple and relatively stress-free was how they survived. The stress in ancient days was different. It was natural. We create our stress from a whole whack of fake.

KEY FACTORS INFLUENCING HEALTH
DIET

We live in a world of extreme. Most people have lost sight of what eating really means, and the necessary connection between your body and mind, required to fulfill your internal nutrition needs.

It comes down to reprogramming your mind to tune into what your body needs nutrient-wise, eating the foods that delivers, and taking repetitive action to ensure you get it habitually. If you don't make these new healthy eating habits stick long-term with a plan, there really is no use.

CIP - Cathy's Important Point - *Life Science, How Stuff Works*, suggests breaking a habit takes 30 days, while creating a new habit takes another 30 days, whereby you're repeating an action systematically and routinely. That's a place to start. Research shows, the longer you repeat an action, the stronger habit it becomes.

I'm not going to get too crazy deep here, but there are a few nutrients in addition to water, 6-8 glasses a day religiously, that your physical body needs to deter disease from setting in, provide energy, build muscle, and transform your body vibrantly strong.

Blunt Talk - Take care of your body, and you decrease your risk of meeting death.
Key Macronutrients and Essential Nutrients
*Lean Protein
*Complex Carbohydrates
*Good Fats (including omega-3s and 6s)
*Essential Vitamins and Minerals

PROTEIN
This is where you might better follow suit of with your ancient ancestors, and eat wild game, and omega-rich fatty fish like salmon. The latter a few days a week. Your mind

needs protein to function, build lean muscle, repair and maintain cells, and promote healthy skin, hair, nails, and bones.

Every cell in your body has protein. It's not stored or manufactured by your body, so you need to get complete protein via food, ideally 2-3 servings per day.
I say complete, because most meats have all the essential amino acids present in the protein to deem it complete. Twenty in total, I think! LOL.

If you're a vegan, and fooling around with dairy sources, beans, and perhaps nuts to get your protein, these are all incomplete. So you're going to have to mix and match, just like a jigsaw puzzle, to make complete proteins. It's an essential move your body needs to break this macronutrient down for energy use.

BEST PROTEIN – Poultry, beef, pork, fish, and wild game, eggs

OTHER PROTEIN – Milk and milk products, beans, nuts and seeds, tofu

*Quinoa is the only plant protein that's complete
When it comes to serving sizes, a piece of meat is approximately the size of a deck of cards, or 4-6 ounces.

For beans, you're looking at ½-3/4 cup. For nuts, it's about a small handful, or 8-10 nuts. 1 egg is a serving. Most of us go way overboard on the serving size. A gynormous factor in our societal obesity issue.
Eating a diverse range of protein with the proper serving size, gives your body the fuel it requires to lose fat sensibly, build sexy lean muscle, or just build your mind and body strong, depending on your health goals.

COMPLEX CARBOHYDRATES

Complex carbohydrates are what your body needs to fuel your systems. When broken down, it's the glucose your body depends on as the primal energy source. This energy is readily accessible and effective.

THE PROBLEM?

Too bad most of us don't know the difference between healthy carbs and bad ones. If you're fuelling your body with a fatty fast-food diet, TV dinners, packaged muffins, cookies, and oodles of chips and sweet treats, you need to read my sugar addiction book, cuz that's exactly what you're fuelling your body and mind with, a gynormous amount of unhealthy sugar.

Sugar does provide energy, but it's short-lived. Simple sugars trigger obesity and disease, like diabetes, cancers, and heart disease. It sends your blood sugar levels for a never-ending roller-coaster ride, triggers depression, and some experts believe sugar's addictive! *Are you kidding me?*

BAD CARBS
*White bread, pasta, and rice
*Pastries, cakes, cookies, and other baked goods
*Chips, candy, chocolate bars, and boxed dinners
***FAST FOOD**, shakes, fries, and greasy burgers

GOOD CARBS
*Whole grain bread, pasta, and rice
*Beans
*Oatmeal, and whole grain breakfast cereals
*Starchy veggies
*Fruits
*Nuts and seeds

Healthy eating choices provide your body with the carbs it requires to function optimally. According to *The Institute of Food and Nutrition*, 6-10 servings per day is optimal. Although, that should be worked out with your nutrition counsellor or medical provider, just to be sure that's the right number for you.

SERVING SIZE
Another area where people get all bunged up, is with the serving size. Doesn't matter what you're eating, if you're eating too much, you WILL get fat!

For bread, it's a slice or ½ of a whole grain bagel. For rice, you're looking at ½ cup, ¾ cup pasta, and the same with beans. One cup of veggies is good. A piece or fruit, or ¾ cup mixed fruit is a serving. ¾ cup of oatmeal or whole grain cereal, is also a serving. A small handful of nuts will do the trick.

We are programmed to eat what's in front of us, not listening to what our body is saying. Try having a little, and if your tummy is still rumbling, have a little more, till you find your balance.

It's a start!

VIP – People overeat because they disconnect their thinking from the physical. We become automated. Eating for comfort, routine, habit, boredom, emotion, and often never consciously realizing how much you've eaten.

This isn't going to change until YOU consciously make the decision to make change, where you consciously listen to your mind and body, in relation to food.

Solution – By keeping a food journal, you'll be shocked into actually seeing how much you really eat each day. This is where your emotions usually get a good smack. Seeing with your own eyes the numbers, all the extra fat and calories YOU shove down your throat, forces you to take ownership.

Sometimes a little negative is necessary to get positive. YOU ARE RESPONSIBLE FOR YOUR OBESITY. This has to be accepted and put behind you, as you take action to make positive eating changes toward better health. The numbers don't lie, and will hold you account-able. For some people, this is exactly what's required to lose pesky fat, and keep it off for good!

GOOD FATS

Without fat, you wouldn't be alive according to *Eating Disorders Online.* Wouldn't it be awesome if we didn't physiologically need fat? And all we had to do to get skinny, was just stop eating it? I think you might want to rub a lamp with that one.

There are two problems with that wishful thinking.
*Your mind and body need fat.
*Obesity is multifactorial. It's caused by social, nutritional, psychological, environmental, physical, and lifestyle fac-tors.

If you want to lose fat, you've gotta commit to addressing multiple factors.

With fats, there's also good and bad choices. The same as with carbohydrates. What makes it even trickier, is that manufacturers are sneaky and hide fats. They have

27

even gone so far as to create a fake or synthetic fat called Trans-fat. This fat is toxic, but cheap, and improves product stability, and shelf life. Packaged processed fatty foods like chips, crackers, and pastries, are prime examples.

Fat Factors
*Provides your body and mind with energy.
*You need fat to help your body absorb fat soluble vitamins, A, D, E, and K.

*It's flavorful, and provides texture and eye appeal to food.
*Satiates hunger longer than other nutrients, which helps control and deter hunger.

*Fat could trigger endorphins in the brain, natural "feel

good" chemicals, just like the ones released after a good workout.
*Not having enough fat may actually cause cravings. Without fat, your body is naturally looking for a way to get satisfied.
*If your blood sugar levels are starved more than 4 hours, fat is your backup energy source to keep your systems running.
*Fat insulates, keeping you warm and snug, and protects internal organs.
*Fat also helps support your organs.
*Nerve impulses run smooth with fat, because it helps to insulate and with transmission.
*Fat is essential in nutrient transport.
*Everything from hormone production to blood sugar levelling, and immune system function, requires fat.
Fat helps you think clearly, heal faster, grow stronger, keep hair and skin vibrant, and keep your overall heath stable and optimal.

Let's have a look at the different fat types.

HEALTHY FATS - Unsaturated

Omega-3 – This is a polyunsaturated fat that helps reduce inflammation, and deter cardiovascular disease.
Sources: Fatty fish like salmon, tuna, mackerel, nuts, pumpkin and flax seeds, oils, olives, and avocados

Omega-6 – Small amounts of this fat is healthy in preventing heart issues. Too much of it triggers your inflammatic response, which is dangerous when these levels are sustained too long. This can result in cancer, arthritis, and heart troubles.

Sources: Nuts, pumpkin, sunflower and flax seeds, oils

Omega-9 – This fat reduces the inflammatory response, reduces the risk of cardiovascular disease, and also reduces the risk of intestinal issues, cancers, and arthritis.
Sources: Nuts, oils
Note - *No oils have all three omegas.*

Monounsaturated – This fat deters heart issues and circulation problems.
Sources: Olives, avocado, sunflower, safflower, corn, and almond oil

UNHEALTHY FATS – Saturated

Saturated – In teeny tiny amounts, sporadically, this fat likely isn't harmful. However, in excessive amounts, like in our society today, saturated fat will increase cholesterol levels, which clogs arteries, and triggers serious disease, like stroke, and heart disease.
Sources: Butter, lard

Trans-Fat – This is synthetic fat that studies show, is a causal factor in cancer and heart disease. Processed food manufacturers use this fat for cost effectiveness, and longevity of food products.
Sources: Packaged and processed foods, fast food burgers and fries, muffins, pastries, and cookies

Cholesterol – Is manufactured from fat in your body, and is found in food. You need cholesterol, but too much triggers cardiovascular disease, and other organ issues.
Sources: Fatty meat, high fat dairy, too many eggs, mac n'cheese, rib-eye steak, ice-cream, liver, and muffins

PHYSICAL EXERCISE

You don't need the *Public Health Agency of Canada* to tell you REGULAR physical activity is critical to good health, well-being, and improved quality of life.

FACTS
*People who exercise regularly live longer, healthier, and happier lives.
*Regular physical activity increases productivity.
*Exercising regularly decreases your risk of injury.
*People exercising have a more resilient immune system.

The human body was physiologically designed to exercise; diverse cardiovascular challenges to build strong your heart and lungs; weight training to strengthen and maintain lean muscle mass for strenuous lifting, pulling, and pushing demands; and stretching to improve agility, mobility, motility, and balance.

In ancient times, elite fitness was necessary for survival; hunting for food, cooking, cleaning, travel, defense, and getting water. Everything our ancient ancestors did required strong muscle, braveness, excellent lung and heart function, flexibility, and agility elite.

Caveman didn't really have a choice whether to drag their tired, achy butt out of bed in the morning. If they wanted to survive, they **HAD** to do it.

Today, it's not instantaneously a life or death situation.

It's not like a hungry lion is going to slip into your house and eat you for breakfast while you lay sleeping soundly. We have the conveniences to get everything we need to survive, without moving a freakin muscle. Our society has automated and digital everything. If you've got the device and the money, you can choose to literally not move a muscle.

Pretty obvious this is a short-circuit-solution-mentality, in which to live. Sure you might be alive, but what sort of quality of life are you living if you are flabby, fatigued, foggy-brained, and infested with chronic illness and disease?

It's a give-take relationship. If you choose not to give your body the intense physical challenges it requires to function optimally; muscles, cardiovascular, stretching and motility, you're on the road to *Dead-Ville*, or at least *Suffer-Ville*.

Tell me something. Why the beep would you knowingly choose that path?

No excuses. It doesn't matter what sort of health issues you're dealing with. There are ALWAYS ways you can fit some sort of physical exercise into your day, within your abilities, that's going to benefit your health.

Just ask your doctor if you don't believe me.

Benefits of Getting Your Motor Running
*Improves weight control
*Decreases the risk of heart disease
*Decreases the risk of cancer
*Improves blood pressure and circulation
*Triggers endorphin release to improve mood
*Taps into hidden energy stores
*Tones the body
*Strengthens muscles and deters injuries
*Speeds up the healing process
*Strengthens immune system function
*Battles the nasty inevitable effects of aging
*Improves overall body function and efficiency
*Betters your mental health
*Gives you a better shot at living longer
*Better overall quality of life
*Less nagging and mood swings

With the support of your healthcare provider, there isn't one single reason you shouldn't be getting your physical on. Sure, it's tough to take the first step.

Suck it up buttercup!
The Answer - Just decide to do it!

Pay attention to your preferences and tolerances, and start slow. Stick with it and turn your biking, walking, swimming, or jogging, into habit over time. Change things up for optimal results, and have supports in place to keep you going. Make sure you've got a plan, chalk full of milestones and rewards. Set your mind to it, and you **WILL!**

Tips to Get Fantastico Physical

The sky doesn't have to be gray, when it comes to routine muscle building, and heart pumping exercise!

Identify your Goals

The first thing you need to do is sit your butt down and write your fitness goals. Do you want to lose weight, tone and strengthen, or make it so you can hike up the stairs without huffing and puffing? Set your timeline too. So you've got a start and finish line that just keeps going. Before you hit the finish line of your first goal, make sure you've got another goal lined up. The mindset here is, gaining momentum. Set a manageable pace that you can sustain forever!

Make a Plan!

If you're going to get serious about pumping more energizing oxygen to your muscles, brain, and hardworking organs, you need to make some sort of plan. Make it a simple open-minded, written down approach, on EXACTLY how you plan to proceed.

Getting help from a trainer is a great way to start, particularly if you're a little rustic creeky-cracky in the body movement department. Your doctor or life coach could also help you with this.

Exercise Plan Considerations are…

*Goals
*Timelines for goals
*Tolerances/preferences
*Physical components – Cardio, muscle building, stretching, core, balance, and agility
*Days of training and times
*Supports in place to pick you up when you fall

33

*Journal to help keep you on track – Other measures?

Focus on keeping it Fun!

Particularly if you've associated negativity with exercis-

ing, it's important to change your thinking. Try looking for the positive. A must if you plan to make your new com-mitment to exercise, stick for life.

If you hate the stinky gym, why not join a bike club that meanders through the trails in the mountains? If you can't

stand swimming, don't do it. Instead, join an intense in-terval training boot camp training session, that maximizes energy expenditure, and minimizes the time spent train-ing.

Brainstorm all the activities you like or could learn to like, and make sure you build your training regimen FUN!

Make it Part of your Day

Exercise training really doesn't do diddly unless you commit to exercising every day as part of your daily rou-tine. Your body needs exercise. It was built to be challenged daily, and you have the sole means to make it happen.

Program it in your phone as a VIP appointment if you have to, and don't be late!

Don't think about it, Just do it!

Particularly when you first start training, there will be times when you just don't want to get your lazy butt out of bed, or you're feeling a tad tired after work, and just don't want to get your sweat on.

It's **WAY** too easy here to make excuses.

Here's where you're best to go into autopilot mode, and just do it without conscious thought.

Particularly if you are exercising first thing in the morning. Set your mind up before you go to bed, that you ARE going to the gym when you wake up. When you rise and shine, don't think about your weary bones and how badly you want to stay cozy under your heavenly covers. Scoot out of bed fast and get to it!

You want to learn to block these negative thoughts, and focus on getting to the gym as fast as you can, before you change your mind. In time, you won't think twice, and you'll just do it!

Supports in Place
It's critical to tell friends and family about your fitness goals. Enlighten them on what your plan is, and that you need them to help keep you on track. Shout it from the mountain top to co-workers, boyfriends, boy-toys, and acquaintances if you like. It's only going to help.

Better still, maybe you can work-out with someone you love. That will increase the odds you'll stick with it. Or perhaps you'll need a trainer that'll crack the whip on you if you're one second late for a forced rep muscle building session?

You know you. Set your supports up accordingly.

WebMD states, having social supports in place when initiating a new fitness program, increases the odds these positive health changes will stick!

Take a Chill Pill

More often than not, you're going to be your worst critic. Take it easy if you happen to go away for the weekend and miss a training session. If you're sick and can't get out of bed for a week, accept it, and let it go. Don't beat yourself up.

The most important factor, is to get back on track ASAP. Focusing on your muck up won't help you get skinny, or reach your running goals. Letting *it* go, and focus forward, more determined than ever to get healthy.

Environment

Your environment both physically and mentally are essential to overall good health. Make sure you're living in a clean environment, free of harmful toxic chemicals, pollution, and any other dangerous substances that could hurt your health.

Just as important, is the fact, you should surround yourself with a positive loving environment. Living with negative energy is going to kill your spirit in time, and most likely your health.

According to a *University of Waterloo* study, individuals immersed in a mentally abusive environment long term, end up with an increased risk of developing both mental and physical issues, compared to those residing in a healthy environment.

There's no doubt stress triggers all sorts of different health ailments. Removing bad or extreme stress, takes away the causal factor, and this act alone can help improve health; mind, body, and soul.

Unhealthy Environments:
*Alcoholics
*Drug addicts
*Gambling or food addiction
*Mental illness untreated
*Sickness in family
*Tragedy, rape, death, terminal illness, and natural disaster
*Financial stress
*Loss of job
*Living in poverty
*Workaholic in the home
*Family member seriously messed up, creating stress
*No normal physical affection in family unit
*No positive family support
*Natural intimate affection is void

*Unhealthy parent relationship – i.e. nasty divorce

Keep in mind, it's all about moderation. A lot of the above

does occur in a healthy environment. It's when issues are ignored or in the extreme, that serious consequences emerge.

Common Feelings to Recognize Negative Environment
*Anger
*Loneliness
*Feeling unappreciated/unheard
*Low self-esteem
*Blamed
*Afraid

*Uncared for
*Sad/depressed
*Feeling dumb
*Disappointment
*Feel like a failure
*Constant worry
*Unable to voice true thoughts
*Anxiousness
*Need for constant attention
*Guilty
*Loss of reality
*Embarrassed about the environment
*The need to be secretive
*Feeling like the black sheep
*Never fitting in
*Loss of control
*Afraid of voicing opinion

These are some of the feelings and beliefs that go hand in hand with a dysfunctional unhealthy environment. The first step is recognizing how harmful your environment is, then build a plan to take action.

Social
Attitudefactor.com states, humans are social animals, and have been since the beginning of time. Our caveman ancestors lived in extended families or tribes, the same thing as apes, which still do.

Historically, when a member of a family is outcast, they usually die. Humans need social interaction for good health.

Scientific studies show, loneliness and negative feelings that manifest, are deadly over time, toxic in nature, triggering disease. Research studies support, that 30 years later, students that were labelled loners or anti-social

growing up, were up to sixteen times more likely to develop cancer, than people venting regularly to friends. Every corner you turn shows clearly that lonely, isolated people, are more likely to attempt suicide, suffer mental illness, participate in high risk activities, get sick more often, and die younger, than the socialite population.
Bottom Line: You need a healthy social life in order to gain optimal health status.

Action Steps:
*Hang out with friends regularly
*Have both romantic and friend/family relationships
*Make time to meet new people and try new activities regularly
In order to lose fat and get healthy, you must get your social life active and balanced.

Mental
When you have control of your emotions, you have good mental health. This includes control of your behavior, enabling you to keep a level head, and handle all the curveballs life throws your way, without going off the deep end.

Typically you bounce back from setbacks faster, and wallow less in misery and despair when you get smacked around some, when you're mentally happy.
What many fail to recognize, is your mental health requires effort and regular maintenance, just like your physical health does.

Taking the time to better your mental will...

*Boost mood
*Build confidence
*Level your thinking
*Decrease moody freakouts

*Enable you to make better decisions, understanding it's physiologically impossible for logic and emotion to tango.
*Increase resilience
*Improve your overall quality and love of life
*Inspire you to want more from life
How you feel about yourself, your ability to control your feelings and handle a crisis, and your ability to maintain quality relationships, are all reflective of your sound mental health.

The aim for fantistico mental health is to ensure…
*Gusto for life
*Happiness with yourself and life direction
*Establishing a sense of purpose
*Ability to have and keep quality relationships
*Maintain balance between work, family, friends, vacation, sleep, and alone time
*High self-esteem
*Belief in your abilities
*Excitement in learning new
*The quick ability to get passed tragedy and back on track positively
*The building of resilience

Action Steps:
-Get stress under control.
-Act positively towards other people. Give compliments because you can. Offer to run errands for someone that can't get out of the house.

-Work at maintaining self-control. When you lose control, is when negative mental health sets in.

-Take the time to go for a walk or just sit in the park and listen to nature. This type of activity is important, proven to help boost natural feel good endorphins in the body, which triggers positive thinking.

-**Work at removing worry.** This one is tough. But working to think positively about yourself and day to day life activities, will only better things.

-**Tap into your senses.** So many times we let external factors interfere and trigger unreasonable thoughts and actions. Use your senses positively, calmly, to boost spirits.

-**Get creative if you can.** Creativity is a form of grounding, which strengthens your mental capacity. You can write, paint, sing, or dance. Pick anything you like to get your creative juices flowing vibrantly.

-**Schedule down time.** Figure out all the things that make you smile from the inside out, and make them a part of your day. Perhaps you like to slip on your headphones and have a nap early afternoon, or go for a roll in the hay, read a great book, or salsa dance?

-**Show gratitude.** By expressing, and tuning into the things you are grateful for each day, you'll strengthen your mind, and overall health too.

My Thoughts…

Your ultimate primal blueprint health is multifactorial. You need to commit to working on better nutrition, exercising daily, finding time for yourself, relationships, mental stress relief, and re-programming your mind positively.

Not an easy task. But if you're serious about finding your body and mental health happiness eternal, you've gotta commit to change, and create a plan to make it reality.

41

42

Chapter 3 – Modern Society Living Issues and Science of Living Basics

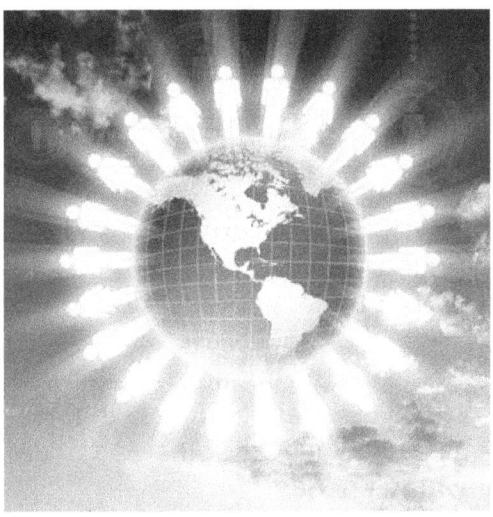

In our fast paced world moving forward at warp speed, we've lost touch with the ancient simplistic factors essential to life and survival:

*Water – Doesn't matter what era you lived in. Your body can't last more than 4 days tops without water. Nutrition experts suggest drinking about 6-8 glasses of water a day in a moderate climate, more if you are exercising strenuously, or living in a sweat box climate.

Dehydration in caveman days didn't typically occur know-ingly. But when water was simply unavailable, man had no choice.

Today, many people become seriously water depleted because they're disconnected with their internal body needs, too busy with life to get off the couch and get hy-drated.

The dangers of dehydration is decreasing your blood vol-ume. It gets thicker. Forcing your ticker to work harder, while less nutrients and oxygen are available to your body.

Consequences of Dehydration are:
*Numbing in fingers and toes
*Less blood to your brain, poorer concentration, and fo-cusing
Carry a water bottle with you, so you stay well hydrated. Avoid drinking soda, coffee, or juices, that just add sug-ars and chemicals to your body, instead of the pure crystal clear water it needs.

*Oxygen – Just a few minutes without oxygen will cause cerebral hypoxia, or brain damage. Shortly after, your or-gans will start shutting down, and then death.
Without oxygen, there is no life.
Smoking and polluted environments reduce the oxygen available, factors our caveman ancestors didn't have to deal with for the most part.

Heart attack and stroke are two health concerns triggered in modern day society, because of poor health choices over time. Each of which, stop oxygen cold from reaching your body.

A few thousand years ago, people might have worried about things like drowning, or perhaps shock from a close call with a wild animal during a hunt. Those were the sorts of things that interfered with oxygen flow. Factors that for the most part are controllable today, but not in days past.

*Nutrition – Water comes first, and then you need sustenance. According to *CBCNews-Health,* the body can go 2-3 days without water, and about 30 days without food.

In dire situations, your body can survive for a limited time on fat stores. Of course this isn't optimal, it just buys time. Without food, your body will use fat. And if your body doesn't have enough protein energy readily available, it will break down your muscles to utilize the protein you've worked hard to make those muscles with, then the glycogen you've got stashed away in your liver. It's a process of complete energy depletion and eventual death.

For about two days, fat reserves are used. Problem is, these fatty acids can't cross the blood-brain barrier, which meaning glycogen from the liver must be utilized for brain function.
Without food, your body shifts into ketosis, energy which can cross the brain-blood barrier, although this only lasts about 2 weeks.

As mentioned previous, when your fat's gone, the muscles are also broken down for energy, lasting no more than a week. Then your body dies.

It is critical for the human body to get adequate daily nutrition for optimal function. If certain essential elements are left out long-term, this triggers the breakdown of good health, cuz a car really doesn't work so well with 3 wheels!

According to *The American Dietary Guidelines*, here's what your body needs each day for optimal health and wellness:
*2-3 servings lean protein
*7-10 servings complex carbohydrates
*2-3 servings healthy fats
*6-8 glasses water

The above gives you an idea of what your body needs daily nutritionally. Which of course varies according to:

-Sex
-Genetics
-Height and weight
-Activity level
-Body composition
-Medical condition
-Lifestyle
-Metabolism

From as far back as we can trace, man has needed these nutritional basics. Nowhere do you see refined sugars, Trans-fat foods, preservatives, dyes, and synthesized chemical elements, that are the main ingredients in many diets today.

These are interference factors, causing sickness and disease, shortened life expectancy, and decreased life quality.

*Sleep – I guess way back in caveman days, people slept because they were tuned into what their body needed.

So physically exhausted by the end of the day, that when the sun went down, sleep was embraced. It wasn't fought and interfered with, which is typical of our society today.

It wasn't until early in the twentieth century that scientists confirmed just how important sleep is for good health. The *American Psychology Association* says sleep is essential to your health and well-being. And that over 40 million Americans, suffer from over 70 different sleep related disorders!

Quality sleep is important. Not getting enough sleep causes temporary and eventual long-term issues. Inadequate sleep lowers body temperature, causes difficulties focusing and concentrating, and triggers hallucinations.

When you don't get the rest your body and mind requires, you lose your cognitive abilities. Sleeping gives your physical body system the opportunity to reset and recharge. Taking that away has the same effect as the pistons being off-time in your car motor. It just won't work correctly.

A minimum 7-8 hours of quality sleep each night is recommended by experts. Although the only way to figure out your magic number, is to set a bedtime and let your body sleep undisturbed through the night, until it naturally wakes, when it's *fully* rested and ready to tackle the day.

*Housing or shelter – Having a shelter helps your body maintain a constant temperature. Of course today, we have clothing to dress appropriately. But hundreds of years ago this wasn't a luxury our ancestors had. It was tough also, because of the physical and environmental restraints.

Without adequate shelter under certain conditions, whole tribes would perish.

FACT - Water loss multiplies when the body is too hot or cold. In the olden days, shelter provided protection, where fire made heat, and the shelter protected from the elements of nature; wind, rain, sleet, ice, dust, and snow. Your normal body temperature is approximately 98.6 degrees F. Hypothermia, or heat stroke, can set in instantaneously without the ability to maintain a constant temperature.

More Facts
-If your body core drops below 91.4, your body goes unconscious.

-Hitting 86 degrees is the ceiling where your body won't be able to regulate temperature.
-Muscles fail at 82.4 degrees F.
-At 107.6 degrees, your central nervous system breaks down.
-A temperature over 111 degrees, triggers your brain to overheat and die.

If you aren't thinking straight, you don't have the ability to make the right decisions to keep yourself alive. Something we take for granted today. Although back in caveman times, it meant certain death.
Secondary factors are, financial status, family, health, and even government function that influence *life*. But these are ever-changing. The bottom line is, without the five factors essential to live, no one person could survive more than a few days.

My Thoughts...

We often take for granted the basic elements for survival, simply because we're spoiled rotten.

A gynormous change from days past, where people were driven daily because of these five elements and working tirelessly to ensure they had the tools to survive. Knowing and accepting that despite their efforts, sometimes Mother Nature would interfere, denying water, animals to hunt, or perhaps triggering extreme weather conditions. The result was certain death.

A HARSH FACT OF LIFE UNCONTROLLABLE!

Our *developed society doesn't have to worry for the most part about getting basic food, shelter, water, oxygen, and sleep, at least to the degree of our resilient ancient ancestors.*

Although one day, the tables just may turn. Something to think about...

Chapter 4 – Primal Blueprint Factor One: Eating: Take Action Pointers

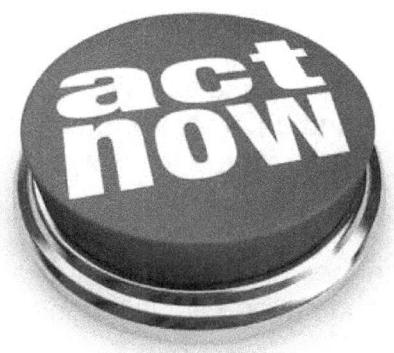

I don't think there's anyone, that doesn't have room to improve on their eating habits. It's not likely you're going to take action immediately, jump in with both feet, and commit to caveman eating and way of life!

It's highly unlikely you've got the horse, spear, or the skills to hunt game, not to mention there isn't much of a game selection roaming freely for you. And the legalities of it aren't in your favor.

I'm being a little silly to make my point. Even if you did want to become a caveman in every aspect, you couldn't.

HIGHLIGHT - This doesn't mean you can't adapt positive eating practices from wholesome and healthy ancient times though.

Modern day society makes it a challenge to choose all natural, pesticide, and hormone-free organic meats, fruits, and vegetables.

Interference Factors - They aren't always readily available, and often expensive.

For instance:
At my local grocery store, a pound of apples is .99, and the same amount of organic apples is $2.49! A bunch of broccoli is $1.49, and an organic bunch is $3.49!
Makes it pretty difficult for me to justify money-wise, feeding my baseball team all-natural!
The idea for establishing your genetic diet, is to make manageable changes one at a time that will stick, transform into habit, and become your new healthy normal.

Action Pointers:
*Minimize Processed Foods
Boxed dinners, packaged muffins and pastries, and greasy fast foods, are loaded with sodium, fat, and added refined sugars. Get into the habit of reading the ingredients. If the list is long and loaded with names you don't

recognize, that's you're signal to drop it and walk away. Just don't do it with your hands up or you're gonna freak people out!

Choose to make your own version from scratch. Instead of buying the Hamburger Helper, why not make your own with whole wheat pasta, lean ground grain fed beef, and your own thickened beef stock. Toss in some chick peas and kidney beans for added fiber.

*Up the Vegetables

Your body can never get enough of the rich vitamins and minerals found in veggies. In particular, vitamin A helps with your immune system function and vision, and vitamin K looks to ensuring bones, joints, and cartilage stay oodles healthy.

The fiber present deters hunger, keeps you regular, and helps you feel satiated longer. Just make sure you're drinking plenty of water. You DON'T want to get constipated.

Veggies are low calories. If you're eating organic or fresh from your garden, you needn't worry about harmful pesticides and toxins. Something that wasn't a concern centuries ago, because crop bug sprays, and hormones to produce higher yields, weren't around.

As natural as possible is best. And frozen is just as beneficial as straight from the organic garden market. When you cook your veggies, don't overdo it. That steals some of the essential vitamins and minerals, which means you aren't getting the best bang for your buck!

6-10 servings per day of fruits and veggies is recommended, for optimal body function. Diversify in the veggies you eat, and pinky swear you'll never shy away from your vegetables.

QUICK TIP – Fill your plate 1/3 veggies, 1/3 complex carbs, and 1/3 lean protein. A great balance when looking to build body strength, blast fat, and gain energy consistently.

*Easy on the Nasty Saturated Fats
This is where our society gets into trouble. Saturated fats like butter and lard, animal fats, and cheese, are **NOT** good for you, particularly in large amounts. Our caveman friends were so active, and got so little saturated fat from the meat they ate, it wasn't much of a concern. The game centuries ago was much leaner for the most part, than the animal our meat sources today.

We seem overdo it, and then some. Loading our potato with ¼ cup saturated butter fat, and a dollop of sour cream. Eating triple cheese pizza like there's no tomorrow. Never mind the pasta dishes with rich creamy sauces, and the warm white simple sugar bread basket we feel the need to drown in butter.

Better choices...
Opt for healthy fats like canola and olive oil for cooking. Get your essential omega fatty acids with some fatty fish, like salmon or tuna, a couple times a week. Ease up on the salad dressing, mayo, and full fat cream cheese. Start by cutting back to half of what you'd normally with saturated fat, then dwindle down from there.

*Choose Mini-Meals
One of the main issues today, is that food is too available, and we just eat **WAY** too much. In order to keep your blood sugars level, moods constant, and energy running strong all day, your body needs healthy fuel regularly. Instead of eating 3 gynormous meals daily, you're best to eat smaller portions more often. So your body's always got accept to readily available energy stores when needed. This also teaches your body to trust, working more effectively at blasting fat while getting you sexy.

*Snack Clean

This one's gonna take a little practice, but it's an important step forward when reversing your eating habits toward caveman style.

First, you need to get rid of all the junk foods in your snack cupboard. The times you do allow yourself a little treat, you'll have to go get it!

This Genetic Diet concept isn't about starving, denying, or depriving yourself. It's about slowly, but surely, changing your thinking and eating habits, to benefit your big picture health.

If your tummy is rumbling between mini-meals, grab a healthy snack. A small handful of nuts, a piece of fruit, or half a whole grain bagel with a smear of peanut butter are great options. Even a whole grain protein bar works in a pinch. Keep these healthy snacks on hand, and don't be afraid to eat smart when your internal systems are calling.

*Detox on the Sugars

Most of us eat **WAY** too many sugars. According to the *American Heart Association*, you don't need more than about 7 teaspoons of sugar per day. By cutting out the juices, sodas, pastries and sweets, you're on your way. Keep in mind. Many breakfast cereals are loaded with sugars, along with yogurts, condiments, and even pasta sauce.

VIP Pointer - Make a habit of reading the labels.
Out with the sugary, and in with the all-natural, will give you control of your health.

*Out with the White!
White bread, pasta, and rice, really do nothing for you.
Loaded with refined sugars and very little nutrients, you'll
gain short term energy, that sends you down to the bottom of the energy barrel fast.

Brown bread, whole grain pasta, and whole wheat rice
are better choices. Loaded with fiber, and ample nutrients
to provide longer term energy, and that important *full feeling* after eating.
Studies show, people that eat whole grains, on average,
weigh less than refined sugar eaters.

*Watch Serving Sizes
Many people *think* they're eating healthy, giving their
body what it needs to fight off those pesky free radicals
looking to trigger disease, but in reality, most people get
too much of a good thing.

Doesn't matter if you are overdosing on fruits and veggies, or forbidden chocolate bars, your body will get fat if
you are consuming more energy than your body is expending.

This is where serving size comes into play.
Restaurant servings are usually at least twice the size
most people need. This means you're getting at least
DOUBLE the lean protein, complex carbs, and healthy
fat your body requires, assuming you are eating healthy.
Your body has no choice but to store this extra energy as
fat, for later use. Re-training your mind and body to know
what a serving size really is, works wonders with your
waistline.

Serving Size Pointers
*A deck of cards, about 4 oz., is a serving of lean meat

*1/2-3/4 cup of beans or legumes
*3/4 cup cooked veggies
*3/4 cup fruit or one piece
*1 slice whole grain bread or half a bagel
*3/4 cup whole grain pasta or whole wheat rice
*1 cup milk
*1/2 cup yogurt
*1 egg or 2 egg whites

*2x2" cube cheese

When you actually look at these serving sizes, please don't have a heart attack. So many people have no idea how much they overeat each meal. Accept and understand this. Then set an action plan to work with the proper serving size for your body.
Your skinny jeans will thank you for it.

VIP NOTE – Back when caveman roamed, they didn't have to pay attention to overeating for the most part. They saw food in a different light, appreciated it because they only ate when Mother Nature was cooperating, and the physical was in place.

They were reactive eatings. When they could, they did. After a feast when the belly was full, they stopped, a form of intermittent fasting many scientists believe helped keep them healthy, lean, and strong.

Today, we eat for so many reasons other than being hungry. This is the problem.
Focus on your eating. Pay attention to what your food tastes like, and listen when your body tells you it's full.
Eat slowly so your body and brain have a chance to signal you to drop the fork.

It's important to know when to stop eating for optimal health and wellness.

*Cravin Sweet – Grab Some Fruit

I'm not talking fruit snacks here, or a piece of bubble berry pie. Fruit is naturally sweet, nicknamed "Nature's Candy," for good reason. You need sugar in your healthy eating plan, but only in moderation.

Fruits like apples, bananas, oranges, and antioxidant loaded berries, provide the energy sugars your brain needs for optimal function. Without all the other crap that comes with processed refined sugars to plug up your system.

Vitamin C and potassium are abundant in both fresh and frozen fruits. Getting at least 3-4 servings per day, will help your internal systems smile. Go for whole pieces of fruit first, because canned fruit in syrup and fruit juices just doesn't cut it.

My Thoughts…

We are looking at two different extremes. The quick and conveniently unhealthy processed way we eat today, and the rustic challenging, and all-natural healthy way of our ancient ancestors.

What's important, is committing to taking steps toward

eating healthier, and more all-natural. It's not about being

perfect, just setting in place changes you can stick to, and love in time.

One change at a time, until you make it habit, is your best route for success.

Commit to better eating. Closer to the way of the cave-man, and you'll reach your health and wellness goals FASTER!

Chapter 5 – Primal Blueprint Factor Two – Exercise – Take Action Pointers

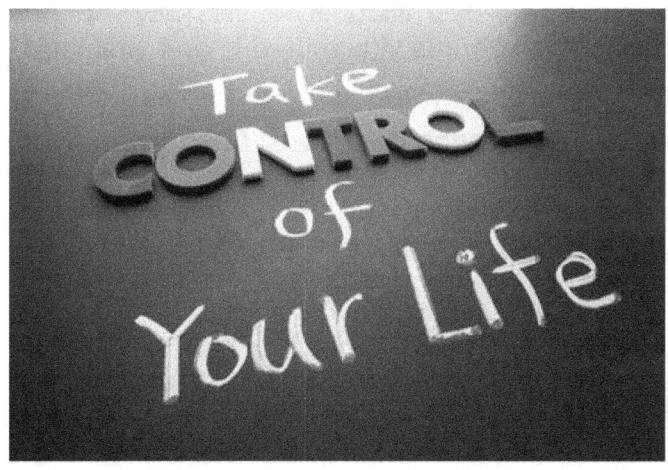

Chances are, you're not conditioned to handle the routine daily physical challenges essential centuries ago. That's okay, we live in a different world today. What is important, is that you take steps to increase the physical energy expenditure in your daily life. It's not something you do once on a blue moon, and except that to suffice.

That just doesn't cut it!
Step by step, you need to incorporate intense cardiovascular, abdominal strength training, stretching, and weights, into your master health and wellness life plan.

Sure, eating healthier helps, but if your body's in physical pristine condition, you're going to reach your fat loss, and optimal health goals oodles faster, not to mention, exercisers long-term, tend to make their fat loss efforts.

STICK!
**This means no more yo-yoing!
According to *The Mayo Clinic*, regular exercise helps control weight, deter disease, increase energy, improve mood, trigger better sleep, pump up the volume with sex, and improve your overall quality of life, how your body processes and absorbs vital minerals and vitamins.

If you still aren't convinced you need to get your butt off the couch, then maybe you should head back into your little cave and **pretend** you're happy.

Take-Action Pointers for Exercise
*Make it Fun

If you don't exercise regularly, or have negative feelings about exercise, it's time to focus on the fun of it! Exercising is work, there is no *automated* when you're sweating up a storm. But it can be fun if you consider your preference and tolerances before you start.

If you are claustrophobic and can't stand the gym, then don't train there. Why not hop on your bike and climb the mountain? And you can always do free weights at home if you prefer. There's group classes, swimming, outdoor bootcamps, gardening, golfing, hiking, and running, as options.

Open your brain and figure out what works for you, instead of focusing on what doesn't, and using that as an excuse!

Figure out what you like or might like to do, and go for it.

If one particular activity doesn't fit, don't use that as an excuse, just try another. Stick with it, and you'll find what works for you.

*Get at Least an Hour in Each Day
Particularly if you are sitting on your fanny most of the day, you need to get your heart and lungs working over-time for at least an hour each day.

Typically experts suggest working your way up to at least 30-45 minutes intense cardiovascular activity each day, and 15-20 minutes weights, and abdominal work 3-4 days.

Of course, stretching should occur before and after every exercise session to help prevent injury.
Understand **ANYTHING** is better than nothing, and you have to start somewhere. Maybe a great goal for you straight off the couch, is to walk around the block at a brisk pace for 20 minutes, do some crunches, pushups, squats, and stretching, and call it a day.

BRAVO for you! My point here, is you need to focus on setting yourself up for success. Make your goals realistic, and climb from there!

If you have little to no experience exercising, I suggest you work with a trainer. This will help you get set up with an effective program, one that will get you results, sup-port your desires, and eventually get you addicted!

*Diversity in Golden
Humans are creatures of habit. Your body loves habit when it comes to pumping your heart and lungs. You see, habit means your body can get lazy. If you do the

same exercise program day in and out, your body will memorize it, and soon just goes through the motions.

Frustrating because you're doing the time, but not getting the results you want, because your mind and physical body are on vacation.

It doesn't take much. Make a point of switching your routine up every couple weeks. Instead of biking for your cardio you could play squash. Use free weights instead of the machines for your weight training, or just do different exercises.

This is also going to help stave off boredom, and ensure you're getting the most out of your sweat time.

*Interval Training Rocks

Hands down, interval training is the most effective way for you to get sexy fit. This maximizes calories burnt, and minimizes time spent training. By alternating periods of high intensity exercise with lower levels, you're going to force both your body and mind to pay attention, burning maximum calories every time.

Incorporating intense weight training with your cardiovascular exercise, is going to push your exercise benefits through the roof.

Without getting into too much detail, muscle burns more calories than fat. And the more lean muscle you have on your body, the more energy you burn at rest.

Bootcamps, cross-training, and circuits, are all excellent interval training routines.
Where no two workout routines are exactly the same. This forces your body to deliver the biggest bang for your sweat bucks.

*Get Support
Having supports in place always helps. Working out with friends or a trainer is a great idea. Talking to your friends and family about your exercise plan, will also increase the odds you stick to it.

*Shut off your Electronic Devices
Seems like we are governed by our smartphones and computers these days. When you're using your devices, that's *sit* time. Make a point of shutting off your electronics and going to the gym, walk the dog, or play pickup basketball with friends.

*Stop Further Away From Your Intended Destination
This works great, particularly if you have an office job in the big city. Park your car a few minutes away from work, to get those endorphins pumping regularly. Just like our caveman friends. Taking the stairs instead of the escalator is another wise move. Or eat lunch on the run, and use your break time for a power walk every day.

In the least, that's going to make your afternoon fly by, with the added bonus of shedding layers!

*Try Something New
Maybe you're used to sitting on your butt after dinner, watching whatever shows have the highest ratings. Commit to trying something new. Like maybe learning how to canoe, go fishing, learn archery, or how about taking some tennis lessons?

Newness is fantastic for your mind, body, and soul. And creating new habits that challenge your muscles and cardiovascular capacity, are golden.

My Thinking…

Regular exercise is a natural component of good health. You need to keep your systems sharp and strong, by getting intense cardio activity and muscle building on a routine basis.

If you need help setting up a program that's going to be beneficial and enjoyable for you, then it's not such a bad idea to hire a personal trainer to get you started on the road to fantabulous health.

The choice is yours. The sooner you get started, the faster you're going to be slim, trim, and living life to the fullest!

Chapter 6 – Primal Blueprint Factor Three – Mental – Take Action Pointers

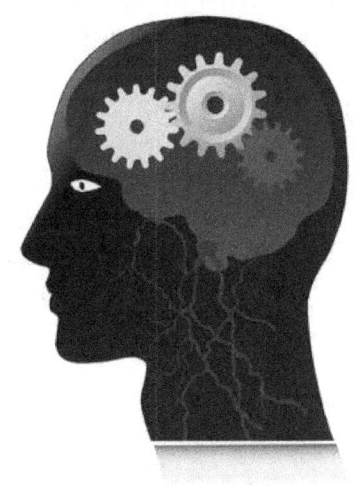

Feeling confident and secure in yourself, is essential for optimal health. How you think reflects both your mental and physical health status. Positive thinking works wonders in setting you up for success in life challenges, making the good better, and the crappy not so bad.
Your mind is a powerful thing.
Your reality is what you believe it to be.

Here are a Few Take Action Pointers to Improve Mental Health
*Make time for things you enjoy

Sometimes the guilt card surfaces. What's important, is setting aside time for things that make you smile. If you love horses, make time to go riding. Perhaps a crossword puzzle in the morning leaves you feeling productive and on the ball!

Look for, and reward yourself with regular bouts of happiness, because this simple mental gift, is reflective of your psychological, and physical well-being.
According to *Michigan University, University Health Services*, taking the time to value yourself, by doing activities you enjoy, helps you find your mental balance. This is critical in your big picture of great health.

*Give Back
It feels good to do things for others. Volunteering your time for causes near and dear to your heart, is a fantastic route to strengthen your mental attitude. Look for ways to contribute to your community, and reap the rewards in the satisfaction for just *doing*.

*De-Stress
I don't care how much of a rock you are, you need outlets to de-stress. I go for a run if my mind is about to explode. Perhaps taking a walk, or even just removing yourself from the situation, and counting down from ten will do the trick.

Make the time to release your stresses daily, or they will stop your momentum, with the intention of one day swallowing you whole.

*Get your Sleep
Not teaching your body to wind down and sleep, adds stress to your life. The body and mind both need to shut

down and recharge nightly. This means getting your zzz's EVERY night, if you want to keep your head on straight. Being tired and groggy doesn't give your mind a fighting chance. Not to mention, sleep deprivation over long periods of time also contributes to serious disease.

Our ancestors didn't have the nightly interference factors society faces in the now, issues that give us excuses to screw up our biorhythms, where our sleep suffers. Artificial lights, all-night clubs, sweet treats within arm's reach, television, smartphones, and all sorts of other electronic gadgets routinely steal sleep.

Ancient people went to sleep when the sun went down, and arose with it. That's the way nature intended it to be. The *American Psychological Association* reports, most heathy adults are built for about 16 hours of wake time. This means 8 hours of quality sleep. Keep in mind everyone is different. There are people that are rested and as quick as a whip, after just 6 hours of zzz's.

*Challenge Yourself
If you snooze, you lose! Experts agree, your mental function naturally degenerates with age. Working your mental helps keep you sharper longer. Crossword puzzles, memory, and brain games, are essential to optimal cognitive function. Your mind naturally wants to be busy. It works like a sponge, and the more new information you feed it regularly, the stronger becomes.

My Thoughts...
These are a few positive mental steps essential when creating your awesome master genetic diet health plan. Your thinking strength helps you implement the positive

health habit changes, required to reach your life health goals.
Train your brain to work harder, and you will be rewarded mind, body, and soul.

Chapter 7 – Primal Blueprint Factor Four: Social/Lifestyle Take Action Pointers

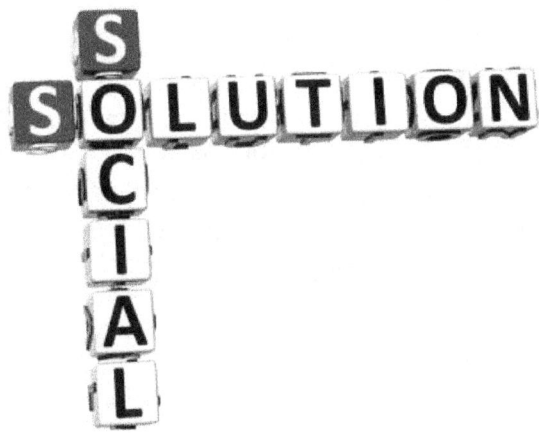

This is where you're going to consider the big picture, each of your life factors that create your lifestyle. This includes the essential social component.
Finding balance in every aspect of your life; physical, emotional, social, and mental, is the ammo you need for you optimal health.

Pointers to Improve your Lifestyle and Social Well-Being
*Strong Connections
Making time to nurture and strengthen family and friend connections, works wonders in keeping your healthy and happy. As humans, strong, trusting, and supportive con-

nections, are essential. This lays the groundwork for persevering through hardship, recovering faster, and refocusing on all that is great.

MailOnline reports academics describe the *Namforsen rock art* discovered in Sweden, as a prehistoric form of Facebook. A social networking system ancient tribes used to learn from one another, evidence humans have always needed social connections.

*Eating Right and Exercising

Of course we've covered both of these aspects. But they're worth mentioning again, because your long-term health and wellness are dependent directly on what you fuel your body with, and how fit you are.

Focusing on smarter food choices, and training your body to build more lean muscle, and increase lung capacity, prepares you to sail through daily life challenges.

Back in caveman times, if the body wasn't nourished and fit, sickness and death resulted. Often life and death decisions, belonged in the hands of fate.

Today, we have control over our physical condition for the most part, and the fuel we use.

It's a matter of committing to positive change.

*Remove Negative Habits

We're well aware, smoking, boozing it up, and using drugs, will eventually kill us in extreme. Unfortunately, each is extremely addictive, making quitting a process. If you're having trouble, seek professional counselling to help you kick your bad habits, opening the door to a clean, healthy lifestyle.

These recreational activities weren't readily available centuries ago. And when they were, life expectancies were so low, that rarely did these negative controllable factors directly cause death.

*Workaholics Die Younger

It's so important for both your mental and physical health, to find balance between work and play. There will always be bills to pay, and chores to attend to. That's never going away. But life will pass you buy faster, if you're not finding things you love to do.

This could be as simple as skipping out of work a few hours early to go for a walk by the water, taking a vacation, checking out a movie flick every month, marking the weekly gals night out in your calendar, or making time to paint, draw, read, or write.

Stop making excuses here, and book *me* time every day.
*Maintenance
This one may seem frivolous, but it's not! Getting your nails or hair done, or heading to the spa for a massage, are activities to improve your overall sense of positivity and appreciation for life. That makes them a priority.

You don't have to spend a lot of money. Just make a point of treating yourself to routine maintenance and pampering, simply because you deserve it.

*Get Happy in Work
Everyone has a choice. If you're not happy in your job, then make a change. There's no use living stressed in your environment, hating your job, and bringing all that negative crap home for everyone else to deal with.

It's your responsibility to yourself, to find a career you are happy in. This reflects positively on everything.

Centuries ago, *jobs* were more or less set in stone, and based around survival. Hunting, cooking, making shelter, gathering firewood, and cleaning, had to be done 24/7, in order to stay healthy and strong. Obviously, times have changed. That doesn't mean you should deny yourself happiness in your occupation.

Forbes reports, finding passion in yourself, helps your head get happy with work!

*Open Your Mind to Change
The clock stops for no one. Your mind needs to change with the times. As new information arises, be open to changing your ways positively. As creatures of habit, humans like to get into a routine, and cement ourselves in. When looking to create your life master plan, this isn't a wise-owl move.

You only know by trying, and excuses just suck. Test out something new and apply if it works. If not, no worries, try something else, till you figure out what suits your lifestyle best.

My Thoughts…
Your lifestyle is an overall reflection of your health in the now, and in the future. With so many more interference factors today, than hundreds of years ago, there's a whole lot more to remove, if you want to live a cleaner lifestyle.

Getting back to the basics is possible. But it's going to take your commitment and time. As always, the choice is yours to make.

Chapter 8 – Myths of Good Eating and Exercise

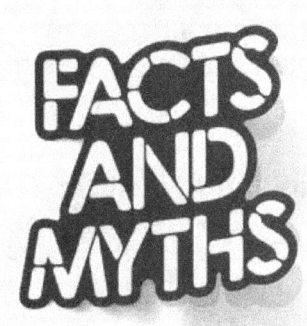

Myth 1: You must load yourself up only with protein after every workout.

Truth – While it's true your body does need protein when exercising, in order to build your muscles strong and rejuvenate energy stores, protein can't do this alone. You also need healthy carbs to provide your hard working body with everything it requires to recover and grow.

Myth 2: Don't eat anything if you train in the morning.

Truth – Now that's a load of hogwash. Do you run your car with no gas in the tank? If you expect your body to perform, you need to provide useable fuel. Even grabbing a banana and glass of milk, or a handful of nuts and an apple, is enough to kick-start your metabolism, and get your body burning clean energy.

Myth 3: Water isn't associated with energy levels.

Truth – The main cause of fatigue when training is dehydration. If you don't keep your fluid levels up, your body won't have the energy it requires to build cardiovascular strength, and create lean muscle mass. Drink water before, during, and after training, to ensure optimal performance.

Myth 4: Get moving and you'll zap fat.

Truth – Effort equals reward. According to *Livestrong* experts, if you are creeping along like a freakin turtle, you aren't going to burn fat. Everybody is different. But good cardiovascular activity should include at least 30 minutes of intensity, pushing your heart rate up to at least 50-85% of your maximum heart rate. A good rule of thumb, is to push yourself hard enough to sweat, but not so hard you can't hold a conversation with someone. If you're training on the cardio machine at the gym, you can track your target heart rate. Just be sure to have a trainer run through it with you. In my experience, these readings are often way out of whack.

Myth 5: If you don't have at least 60 minutes to train, don't bother.

Truth – With just 15-20 minutes of high intensity interval training, HIIT, you can reach your fitness goals and beyond. Don't be afraid to break your training sessions up.

This works well when you're running short of time, and encourages your body to burn more fat and calories as a whole. It also works to boost your metabolism up longer, after you've finished training.

Keep in mind, it's not necessarily the time you spend training that's important, but rather the number of sweat buckets you collect.

Myth 6: Cutting carbs is going to make you super skinny.

Truth – That'll leave you grouchy, hormonal, and weak.

Your body needs carbs. What's important, is ditching the simple sugar processed white carbs; cake, cookies, pastries, chips, sweets, white bread, and fast foods; and adopting healthy vitamin packed whole grain breads, brown rice, and whole wheat pasta, legumes, and veggies.

Don't starve your body. Get the 6-10 servings of healthy carbs you need each day, and give your body the means to blast fat.

Myth 7: If you're injured, don't exercise

Truth – In most instances, with a few modifications, you can, and should continue to train. Of course, check with your doctor. But if you have a minor tear or strain, it's quite simple to just work around the injury. And often you can still work your injured area, just take it easy, and don't work it to full capacity.

This helps you stay in the groove, recover faster, and often come out stronger than before the injury.

Final Words

We are totally spoiled with convenience and technology. Removed from our world are the basic needs for survival our ancient ancestors had to fight for daily. We don't have to rise with the sun to hunt game for breakfast, battle the elements of nature, and trek 5 miles uphill for water.

In actuality, we don't even have to lift a finger to get the basics. Well maybe a finger. You can dial up the local pizza shop for food, bribe your boyfriend to bring you some water from fridge water dispenser, and when it comes to shelter, you can just buy or borrow one.

We don't naturally get the daily muscle building and cardiovascular challenges cavemen did. Many of the food choices we make are fake, processed, synthetic, and loaded with bad carbs, sugars, sodium, and unhealthy fabricated Trans-fats.

Instead of dealing with stress by exercising or becoming one with nature, we learn to grab a tub of triple chocolate ice cream, and drown our stresses with a sappy movie. Instead of releasing, we store them away. This increases our internal tension, so eventually it explodes. It can surface as a mental or physical sickness.

Our unhealthy lifestyles of too much fatty food, not enough exercise, dysfunctional relationships, not enough natural *fight or flight challenges*, and external stresses from work, family, our environment, and unhealthy life-styles, all contribute to poor health.

All of this, makes it incredibly difficult to focus of the bare bones basics of what we need to survive, and what you need to be happy.

What is your balance?
Do you really need that fast food burger, fries, and a shake? Or could you get used to barbecuing a grass fed organic burger, on a whole grain bun, with grilled sweet potato, and fresh squeezed orange juice?

Would it be so bad to trade in your video games for a bike, and sell one of your old smartphones for some free weights?

How about changing your daily regimen to get your butt out of bed an hour earlier, to get your heart and lungs working before you plunk yourself down behind your desk for the day?

One thing for certain is, by getting back to the basics, your body will have no trouble zapping fat and growing lean, strong, beautiful sexy muscle. Cutting out pro-cessed foods, eating less, choosing nutrient rich foods in proper amounts, including intense cardiovascular and weight lifting interval exercising, while implementing posi-tive mental, social, and lifestyle change, is only going to boost your love for life, and increase the quality in which you live it.

Our ancient ancestors, the caveman, didn't have the

choices of luxury we have today. They weren't afraid of a lot of hard work just to keep their bellies full, bodies warm, strong and fit, and keep disease away.

You have choices, and if you are serious about creating your master primal blueprint diet. All you have to do is commit to **TAKE ACTION**.

I'm just curious…Do you think you could handle it cave-man style?

Last Thoughts…

*THANK-YOU for reading my masterpiece. I hope you learned a little something, or at least got a few smiles.
*I would appreciate a millisecond or three of your time for a quick review, to help me build my masterful book empire higher.
*Whatever you do, don't forget to smile, and of course, check out my website for more of my e-Book masterpieces! www.flawlesscreativewriting.com

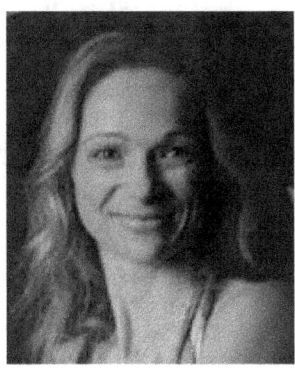

Cathy☺

Disclaimer

www.ingramcontent.com/pod-product-compliance
Lightning Source LLC
Chambersburg PA
CBHW070558290526
45790CB00002B/728